Traumatic Brain Injury in the United States: The Future of Registries and Data Systems

Summary and Recommendations from the

Expert Working Group

Atlanta, Georgia

July 1–2, 2002

Prepared by:

Division of Injury and Disability Outcomes and Programs

National Center for Injury Prevention and Control

Centers for Disease Control and Prevention

U.S. Department of Health and Human Services

June 2005

Traumatic Brain Injury in the United States: The Future of Registries and Data Systems

This report is a publication of the National Center for Injury Prevention and Control, Centers for Disease Control and Prevention.

Centers for Disease Control and Prevention

Julie Louise Gerberding, MD, MPH

Director

National Center for Injury Prevention and Control

Ileana Arias, PhD

Acting Director

Suggested Citation: Langlois JA, Rutland-Brown W. Traumatic Brain Injury in the United States: The Future of Registries and Data Systems. Atlanta (GA): Centers for Disease Control and Prevention, National Center for Injury Prevention and Control; 2005.

Editors

Jean A. Langlois, ScD, MPH

Division of Injury and Disability Outcomes and Programs

National Center for Injury Prevention and Control

Wesley Rutland-Brown, MPH

Division of Injury and Disability Outcomes and Programs

National Center for Injury Prevention and Control

Acknowledgements

The editors wish to acknowledge the valuable contributions of the following people to the meeting on the Future of Traumatic Brain Injury Registries and Data Systems and to the production of this report: Doug Browne, Jacqui Butler, Michelle Huitric, Angela Marr, Jane Mitchko, Teri Ricker, and the staff of the Office of Communication Resources, National Center for Injury Prevention and Control, CDC.

The reason for collecting, analyzing, and disseminating information on injuries is to control those injuries and their effects.

Collection and analysis should not be allowed to consume resources if action does not follow.

— adapted from William H. Foege, Former Director, Centers for Disease Control and Prevention, 1976.

Group Participants

Christine Baggini
Director of Family Resources
Brain Injury Association of Virginia
Richmond, Virginia

Allan Bergman
President and CEO
Brain Injury Association of America
McLean, Virginia

Susan Connors
Executive Director
National Association of State
 Head Injury Administrators
Bethesda, Maryland

John Corrigan, PhD
Professor
Department of Physical
 Medicine and Rehabilitation
Ohio State University
Columbus, Ohio

Thom Delilla
Bureau Chief
Brain and Spinal Cord Injury Program
Florida Department of Health
Division of EMS and Community Health
 Resources
Tallahassee, Florida

Lt. Betty Hastings
Director
Traumatic Brain Injury Program
Maternal and Child Health Bureau
Health Resources and Services Administration
Rockville, Maryland

Jean A. Langlois, ScD, MPH (Moderator)
Senior Epidemiologist
Health Outcomes and Disability Prevention
Division of Injury and Disability Outcomes
 and Programs
National Center for Injury Prevention and
 Control
Centers for Disease Control and Prevention
Atlanta, Georgia

Dave Murday, PhD
Assistant Director
Center for Health Services & Policy Research
University of South Carolina
 School of Public Health
Columbia, South Carolina

Anne Rohall, Esq
Director of Government Relations
Brain Injury Association of America
McLean, Virginia

Pat Sample, PhD
Associate Professor
Department of Occupational Therapy
Colorado State University
Fort Collins, Colorado

Karen A. Schwab, PhD
Statistician
Defense and Veterans Brain Injury Center
Uniformed Services University of the
 Health Sciences
Bethesda, Maryland

Anbesaw W. Selassie, DrPH
Assistant Professor
Department of Biometry and Epidemiology
Medical University of South Carolina
Charleston, South Carolina

Mary Stuart, ScD
Chair
Department of Sociology and Anthropology
University of Maryland, Baltimore County
Baltimore, Maryland

Michael Weinrich, MD, PhD
Director
National Center for Medical Rehabilitation
 Research
National Institute for Child Health and
 Development
National Institutes of Health
Bethesda, Maryland

Table of Contents

Executive Summary

This report summarizes the comments, suggestions, and recommendations of a working group convened by the Centers for Disease Control and Prevention (CDC) to discuss the future of traumatic brain injury (TBI) registries and data systems. It is intended for policy makers, researchers, advocates, and public health professionals, including those from state health departments, interested in furthering the development of systems to collect data about people with TBI and to help those people learn about available services such as health care, employment training, and personal assistance.

In the Children's Health Act of 2000, Congress authorized CDC to develop a "National Program of TBI Registries" to collect data about TBI. Currently, CDC supports other TBI data collection systems, including TBI surveillance, that can also be used to identify people with TBI and help them get information about services.

On July 1–2, 2002, CDC convened an expert panel of TBI researchers, advocates, registry administrators, and other professionals to discuss the future of TBI registries and data systems and to obtain guidance in the development of a "National Program of TBI Registries."

Meeting participants first reviewed background information about registries and existing CDC-funded TBI and injury data systems, including TBI surveillance. Second, they developed a simple working definition of a TBI registry and described its key functions:
- Collect TBI data;
- Identify people who sustained a TBI (maintaining personal identifiers and contact information);
- Link people with TBI to needed information and services.

Third, the panel used this definition as a framework to discuss whether TBI data systems, such as surveillance, might serve the important functions of a registry. Finally, they recommended ways that CDC could enhance currently funded TBI data systems to build TBI registries.

The expert panel members noted that TBI registries do provide useful information about TBI in some states. However, because of the CDC's prior work in developing and implementing standard population-based data collection (surveillance) in most states and the greater cost of implementing most registries, they agreed that the expansion of state-based TBI data collection efforts could best be facilitated by expanding and enhancing existing TBI and injury surveillance data systems. They also recommended that CDC place a high priority on developing state-based data systems that can help link people with TBI to needed information and services. Meeting participants also recommended a wide range of other activities that would enhance TBI research and programs.

Background

The Future of Traumatic Brain Injury (TBI) Registries and Data Systems

Purpose of the Report

On July 1–2, 2002, the Centers for Disease Control and Prevention (CDC) convened an expert working group to discuss "The Future of TBI Registries and Data Systems." This report documents the group's comments and suggestions.

Meeting Goals and Objectives

CDC convened the meeting to obtain guidance in responding to new language in the Children's Health Act of 2000, which charged the agency with developing a "National Program of TBI Registries." (See text box, pg. 6, for details about legislation authorizing CDC's TBI activities.)

There were several objectives for the meeting:

- Develop an operational definition for the term *registry*;
- Discuss how CDC's current TBI data collection activities might serve as the basis for developing a new registry;
- Recommend future CDC activities.

Meeting Participants and Process

The 13 participants included TBI researchers, advocates, registry directors, and representatives from state and federal government agencies. With input from the Brain Injury Association of America (BIAA), the National Association of State Head Injury Administrators (NASHIA), and the National Institutes of Health (NIH), CDC selected invitees based on their experience and potential to contribute to a greater understanding of the need for TBI data systems, such as registries, and the best approaches to developing state-based data systems. At the time of the meeting, two participants were involved in managing state-based TBI registries in Florida and Virginia; one participant was the principal investigator for both a CDC-funded statewide TBI surveillance system and a TBI follow-up registry in South Carolina.

For the first two objectives, CDC staff prepared background material for discussion, including a draft definition of a registry and an overview of CDC's current TBI data collection activities. The meeting began with an overview of this material, followed by presentations by meeting participants who were directly involved in managing TBI registries or surveillance systems. These participants presented information about their programs and answered questions. For the remainder of the first day, participants discussed the information from the background presentations. A professional note taker recorded participants' comments and suggestions. On the second day, the moderator presented a synthesis of the suggestions for review and revision by the participants.

This report documents the final summary of comments and recommendations by working group members. For some sections, more detailed information, references, and other materials have been added to clarify and update the information presented at the meeting.

Readers of this report should also consult the companion website, Traumatic Brain Injury Data Collection at www.cdc.gov/ncipc/profiles/tbi. This site provides detailed information about state-based TBI data systems, including those discussed at the expert meeting.

Summary of Presentations

CDC staff and selected meeting participants presented the following background information:

The Need for TBI Data Systems or "Registries"

According to national statistics, more than one million people in the United States survive a traumatic brain injury each year, and at least 80,000 of them experience long-term disability as a result of their injuries (Thurman et al. 1999).

Before states can adequately respond to this important public health problem, each state must determine the number and characteristics of people affected, categorized by age, sex, race, etc. Registries in Florida and Virginia, for example, have proven useful for this purpose; many other states have successfully used various other approaches to collecting information about people with TBI. Regardless of the approach, advocates, policy makers, and TBI service providers agree that TBI data must be specific to each state to effectively inform primary prevention activities, policy development, and planning to ensure adequate services for people with TBI.

The Children's Health Act: CDC's Charge to Develop TBI Registries

Each state needs TBI information about its residents. Recognizing this need, Congress, in the Children's Health Act of 2000, authorized CDC to develop a "National Program of TBI Registries." The objective is for CDC to "make grants to states to operate the state's traumatic brain injury registry...to collect [TBI] data... about the demographics and clinical characteristics of persons hospitalized with TBI." (See text box, pg. 6, for details about legislation authorizing CDC's TBI activities.)

Legislation Authorizing CDC's TBI Activities

The TBI Act of 1996 (PL 104-166)

In 1996, the U.S. Congress passed Public Law 104-166, the Traumatic Brain Injury Act. This Act required CDC to:

- Further develop uniform TBI reporting systems among states;
- Submit a report to Congress about TBI incidence and prevalence (National Center for Injury Prevention and Control 1999b).

  (For actual language, go to http://thomas.loc.gov/bss/d104/d104laws.html. Select the range 104-151 to 104-200 and click search. Scroll down to 166. Select text or pdf.)

The Children's Health Act of 2000 (HR 4365)

In 2000, Congress passed TBI Act amendments which required CDC to:

- Disseminate national information on the incidence and prevalence of TBI.
- Provide information in primary care settings concerning the availability of state-level services.
- Develop a national education and awareness campaign.
- Develop a National Program for TBI Registries. Make grants to states for operating the state's traumatic brain injury registry and collect data such as the following:

  ○ Demographic information;
  ○ Circumstances of injury;
  ○ Source of the information, dates of hospitalization and treatment, date of injury;
  ○ Information characterizing clinical aspects of the injury, including types of treatment and services used.

(For actual language, look at Title XIII – Traumatic Brain Injury at http://thomas.loc.gov/cgi-bin/bdquery/z?d106:HR04365:. Select text or pdf.)

Registries or Surveillance?

Considerations in Implementing the Children's Health Act

Background

Registries do provide useful data about TBI in some states. However, several factors should be considered in determining the best approach to developing a national program of TBI registries. First, as of January 2005, CDC supports injury data collection systems in more than 30 states, including TBI surveillance in 11 of these states. Second, although the need for national data on the impact of TBI in the United States is often used to support the need for a national registry system, CDC has routinely and successfully used existing national data sets maintained by the National Center for Health Statistics to meet that need (Thurman et al. 1999). Third, although not specifically stated in the authorizing language, CDC supports the idea that where possible, TBI data systems should also provide information about the outcomes and service needs of people with TBI and link those individuals to needed services, such as personal assistant services, transportation, or help finding employment. TBI service agency staff, advocates, and other professionals also support this view. Finally, in addition to duplicating other data collection efforts, the development of a program of registries separate from current CDC data collection efforts could be very costly. CDC is charged with conducting a wide range of other TBI-related activities with limited funding totaling approximately $5.7 million in FY 2005.

What Is a Registry?

General Definition

A registry can be defined as "a collection of data about a particular group of people who share a common personal characteristic, for example development of the same disease…" (Feinstein 1998, p.475). However, there is wide variation in the type and nature of registries, which can range from a simple list of people affected by a disease or condition, to a complex system of identifying, contacting, and providing case coordination to help people with the condition get the services they need.

Characteristics and Functions of a TBI Registry

The expert panel members discussed the following background information about registry functions and funding mechanisms.

- Data collection

  TBI registries vary in the type and completeness of the data collected. Collecting data about people who experience a TBI is the most basic function of a registry. TBI registries typically collect information about demographics (e.g., age, sex, race), clinical characteristics (e.g., the type and severity of the injury to the brain), and the external cause of the injury (e.g., fall, motor vehicle crash). Data about other factors that can influence recovery (e.g., the presence of other health conditions) are sometimes collected.

- Identification

  A key feature of a registry is legal authority to identify people with the condition and maintain and use their personal identifying information to contact them. Contact is usually initiated to request their enrollment in research studies or to provide them with helpful information about available services. TBI registries typically identify patients soon after they are admitted for medical care.
  The registries usually require specialized staff to review medical records and either enter the data into a special data system or forward the data to another location for management. This allows for early identification of people with the condition, ease of tracking them over time because accurate contact information is obtained, and flexibility in the amount and type of data collected. However, unless extensive resources and rigorous methods are applied, the reporting of cases is often incomplete. Such a registry can also be costly. For example, CDC provides about $35 million per year to fund operation of state cancer registries (personal communication: P.M. Talboy, CDC, 2002). Each state also contributes funding to support this activity. (See the CDC National Program of Cancer Registries website: www.cdc.gov/cancer/npcr.)

- Linkage to services

  Helping link people with TBI to services is an important function of a TBI registry, according to experts in the field (National Center for Injury Prevention and Control 1999a). Assistance in obtaining services is particularly important for people with TBI because cognitive problems resulting from their injury make it difficult for them to find and access the services they need to compensate for these problems (General Accounting Office 1998).

- Follow-up data collection

  Contacting and interviewing people with TBI to find out about the nature and extent of the problems they experience as a result of their injury can help increase knowledge about the factors that influence recovery and the services these people need. TBI often results in long-term disability that interferes with performance of routine daily tasks, return to work or school, and successful community reintegration (National Institutes of Health 1999). Quantifying these problems can provide information needed by state agencies to plan for and justify funding for the services that residents with TBI need.

- Funding

  Most TBI registries currently rely heavily on state funding dedicated to supporting the registry, including some that receive funding from trust funds, for example from fines for driving under the influence.

Examples of TBI Registries

The following is a brief summary of basic information about selected TBI registries.

States

The Florida Brain and Spinal Cord Injury Program (FBSCIP) supports a TBI and Spinal Cord Injury (SCI) registry that identifies moderately to severely injured people with TBI while they are still in the hospital. The program focuses on case management to facilitate coordination and payment for rehabilitation services needed for their return to the community. Florida residents with mild TBI also have access to assistance through contractual services with the Brain Injury Association of Florida and special projects (personal communication: K. Shields, FBSCIP, June 2004). The staff of the Florida registry indicated that all people hospitalized for moderate to severe TBI are routinely reported to the registry (personal communication: T. DeLilla, FBSCIP, July 2002). (See the Florida Brain and Spinal Cord Injury Program website: www.doh.state.fl.us/Workforce/BrainSC.)

Virginia operates a TBI/SCI registry in which hospitals report information about new cases of TBI/SCI to a centralized data center at discharge (personal communication: C. Baggini, Brain Injury Association of Virginia, July 2002). Individuals of all ages who are treated for mild, moderate, or severe injuries, including those treated and released from a hospital emergency department, are expected to be reported to the registry. Outreach material is sent to those who are reported, and subsequent information and referral services are provided to those who request them. Not all hospitals report all cases to the Virginia registry (personal communication: C. Baggini, Brain Injury Association of Virginia, July 2002). Although reporting to the Virginia Central Registry for Brain Injury and Spinal Cord Injury is mandated by the Code of Virginia, there are no sanctions available to ensure compliance. This is a common problem for registries that cannot enforce hospital reporting and for which funding is limited. (See the Virginia Central Registry website: www.biav.net/central_registry.htm.)

The exact costs of operating registries are difficult to calculate because various tasks may be performed by different agencies, facilities, or personnel. The Florida TBI registry relies on funding from the Brain and Spinal Cord Injury Rehabilitation Trust Fund. Florida estimates the cost of TBI data collection only (excluding case coordination and other registry functions) at $75,000 per year. The Virginia registry is supported by state funding. Virginia's costs for TBI data collection only are reported to be approximately $125,000 per year.

Military

The Defense and Veterans Brain Injury Center (DVBIC) supports a registry and tracking system that identifies and follows consenting military personnel and veterans who were diagnosed with and treated for a TBI. Clinicians in designated facilities, including three military medical centers, four veterans' affairs medical facilities, and one civilian community reentry facility, are asked to report all people hospitalized with a TBI to a central registry. Medical centers also collect information about patients treated and released from emergency departments and outpatient clinics. An important function of the registry is to help people with TBI obtain appropriate services, receive follow-up clinical contacts, and receive appropriate educational materials. (For more detail see: www.dvbic.org.)

Working Definition of a Registry: Key Registry Functions

Based on the information presented previously, the expert panel concluded that the working definition for a TBI registry should include the following primary functions (also shown in Figure 1):

- Data collection;
- Identification (maintaining personal identifiers and contact information), considered a key function that distinguishes a registry;
- Linking people to services (helping them get information about available services).

Figure 1. Model for Building TBI Registries

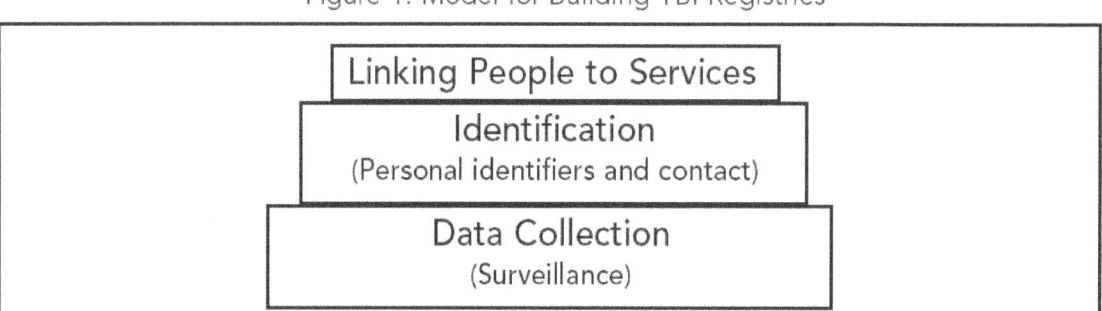

Figure 1 illustrates the potential for registry systems to be built on existing TBI data collection systems (shown at the base of the figure) by adding to the basic data collection function the functions of identification and linking people to services.

Three secondary functions were considered:

- Data linkage: Linking registry information to data from other sources, such as Medicaid claims data, in order to track the use of social services and related costs. Including in the data system personal identifiers such as social security numbers can facilitate such linkages.
- Follow-up data collection: Contacting people who have had a TBI and interviewing them to find out about health and other problems they may be experiencing.
- Evaluation: Evaluating whether people with TBI who were linked to services were satisfied with the services and benefited from them.

Other Data Systems

In addition to the registries described previously, other state-based data systems have proven useful or shown the potential to provide needed information about TBI. The primary sources of state-based TBI data are described below.

TBI Surveillance

TBI surveillance is the most promising data system that could be enhanced to serve the functions of a TBI registry. For that reason, the description of surveillance by registry function (below) is more detailed than that of the other data system mentioned. Additional information about TBI surveillance is available in the article "Traumatic Brain Injury-Related Hospital Discharges" (Langlois et al. 2003), from this report's companion website about TBI data systems (see data systems website: www.cdc.gov/ncipc/profiles/TBI), and in the *CDC Annual CNSI Data Submission Standards* (Marr and Coronado 2004).

- Data collection

Definition and description of TBI Surveillance

Surveillance is defined as *routine, ongoing collection of data about people who sustained a TBI*. States that conduct TBI surveillance process and analyze TBI data obtained primarily from statewide mortality data sets and existing administrative data sets, including statewide hospital discharge data sets that were originally developed for billing purposes. Thus, TBI surveillance differs from most registries because it does not require a dedicated hospital-based system for collecting data about people hospitalized with TBI. As a result, surveillance also has the advantage of being low cost in relation to the completeness of case ascertainment and the quality and extent of the data obtained. As of January 2005, CDC funded 11 states to conduct TBI surveillance. Each state received $80,000 per year to process basic data about the number and demographics of people hospitalized with TBI in their state. Six of these states also received $65,000 to abstract additional information from medical records.

TBI registries and surveillance vary in the extent to which they capture all cases of TBI that occur within a state. Despite some limitations in case identification, CDC-funded TBI surveillance tends to have more complete case identification than TBI registries because surveillance data are routinely collected for billing purposes. Thus, surveillance data are described as *population-based*; that is, these data include all or nearly all of the hospitalized TBI cases in a geographically defined area (or state), allowing for an accurate assessment of the impact of TBI in that area. Ideally, TBI registries should also be population-based. However, even with state mandates, many registries underreport TBI cases. (See text box, pg. 17, for additional information about population-based data systems.)

Limitations of data collection using TBI surveillance

- Timeliness

  TBI surveillance states vary in the amount of time required to obtain the administrative data sets. The average time is currently 12 to 18 months after the close of the calendar year.

- Flexibility

  Because most states use existing administrative data sets, the information that can be collected is limited to what is already routinely collected. Some state surveillance systems abstract additional information from hospital records, but that information is limited to what is recorded.

- Completeness of case ascertainment

  Although considered to be population-based, the TBI surveillance system does not capture "all" cases. For example, because most state surveillance systems funded by CDC collect only data on deaths and hospitalizations, people with TBI who are not admitted to a hospital are not included.

Even states that collect data on people who are treated and released from the ED will miss those who do not seek and receive medical care or who are seen by private doctors.

State-based hospital discharge data systems frequently miss people treated in prison hospitals, military and veterans' hospitals, Indian Health Service hospitals, or hospitals in another state. However, these omissions typically result in a relatively small percentage of hospitalized cases that are not identified.

- Availability of data

  States vary in the kind and amount of TBI data that are available. Some state data systems have missing cause of injury codes (E codes) for a large proportion of data; E codes describe, for example, whether an injury resulted from a fall or motor vehicle crash.

- Identification

  Some states with TBI surveillance have legal authority to identify and contact people with TBI that reside within the state. This allows states to collect and keep information such as names and addresses within the surveillance data set for collecting follow-up data or linking them to services.

- Linkage to services

  TBI surveillance systems in states with legal authority to identify and contact people with TBI can serve an important role in linking state residents with TBI to information about available services. With CDC funding, the Colorado Department of Health and the Environment, in collaboration with the Colorado State University, the Brain Injury Association of Colorado, and the Colorado HRSA-funded TBI services project, investigated whether surveillance system data could be used to help link people with TBI to services. Using their legal authority, the Colorado TBI Surveillance Program identified from the surveillance system a sample of people hospitalized with TBI.

Project staff then sent them letters about a new 800 number with information about available services. This effort resulted in a fourfold increase in the number of calls to that number (personal communication: P. Sample, Colorado State University, 2002).

These efforts demonstrate the potential for TBI surveillance to be used to help people with TBI find out about and access needed services. As of January 2005, an evaluation of the effectiveness of the 800-number project to find out whether people with TBI who called the number actually got the services they needed is in progress.

- Other functions

Follow-up data collection

Colorado and South Carolina have conducted multiyear follow-up studies of a representative sample of people with TBI in their states. Specifically, they successfully contacted a sample of people identified through surveillance and interviewed them by telephone to learn about their TBI-related problems and service needs (Brooks et al. 1997; Pickelsimer et al. 2002) (See the South Carolina Traumatic Brain Injury Registry website: sctbifr.musc.edu.)

Core Injury Surveillance

As of January 2005, CDC funds 28 states for injury surveillance. These programs must have the ability to access and analyze injury data sets recommended by the State and Territorial Injury Prevention Directors' Association (STIPDA 2003). The Core injury programs categorize and analyze injury data by external cause (e.g., motor vehicle crashes, falls). However, because many of the data sets used for Core injury surveillance are the same as those used for TBI surveillance, analysis of TBI data by these programs is feasible. Some states, including Massachusetts, include analysis of TBI data as part of this effort, and some report basic TBI rates as part of the State Injury Indicators project in which CDC staff, in collaboration with members of the State and Territorial Injury Prevention Directors' Association, advise states on the methods for calculating rates of injury, including TBI. (See the Indicators website: www.cdc.gov/ncipc/pub-res/indicators.)

These efforts show the potential for existing injury surveillance and other data collection efforts to form the base for expanding TBI surveillance to other states because the states involved in Core injury surveillance or the Indicators project already have access to the basic data needed for TBI surveillance. By 2006, CDC anticipates that all states participating in Core injury surveillance will analyze and report separately their data for TBI. (See the Core State Injury website: www.cdc.gov/ncipc/profiles/core_state.)

Definition of Population-Based

"Population-based" is an epidemiologic term describing a registry or other data collection system that has information about "all" cases of a specific disease or injury in a geographically defined area that relates to a specific population. For example, the population-based TBI surveillance system in Colorado identifies each year all state residents hospitalized with TBI within the state whose billing information is included in the statewide hospital discharge data set. However, population-based does not mean that everyone who has ever had a TBI is included in the registry or surveillance data set.

- Population-based TBI registries and surveillance systems typically focus on hospitalized cases; therefore, they provide population-based data only about the TBI population that is hospitalized.
- People who were injured before the system was established, those not admitted to the hospital, persons who were misdiagnosed, and those for whom the TBI diagnosis is missed (including people with other more severe injuries or health conditions) are not routinely included in registries and surveillance systems reporting only about persons hospitalized.
- Some registries with the primary goal of helping people get services identify cases in other ways, for example by allowing self-reported cases, demonstrated by the Defense and Veterans Brain Injury Center's registry. The advantage of this type of registry is that more people can benefit from potential linkages to services, and more information on the prevalence (the number of people living with TBI-related problems) may be obtained. A disadvantage is that accurate information about the injury—for example, a clinical assessment of the severity of the TBI—is lacking for self-reported cases.

Recommendations of the Expert Panel

Following the presentations and discussion summarized above, expert panel members agreed upon the following recommendations.

General

At both the state and national levels, CDC should continue to support and conduct activities to collect, analyze, and use population-based TBI data and data systems:

1. To determine

   - Incidence and prevalence of TBI-related disability and trends over time;
   - External causes of and risk factors for TBI;
   - Outcomes of TBI including information about the natural history of recovery;
   - Service needs of people with TBI.

2. To help link people with TBI to information about

   - Traumatic brain injury in general, including what to expect during recovery;
   - Available services.

CDC should place a high priority on developing state-based data systems that can help people with TBI get needed information and services.

Developing a National Program of TBI Registries

The expert panel noted that TBI registries provide useful information about TBI in some states. However, because of the CDC's prior work in developing and implementing standard population-based data collection (surveillance) in the majority of states and the greater cost of implementing most registries, they agreed that the expansion of state-based TBI data collection efforts could best be facilitated by building on existing TBI and injury surveillance data systems. States with legal authority to identify and contact people with TBI could enhance these systems to add functions such as linkage to services or follow-up to find out about TBI outcomes.

Specific recommendations for implementation at state and national levels follow:

Data Collection

- State level

1. CDC should fund more states to collect, analyze, and report TBI data.

   ◦ CDC should work to make sure all 50 states, the District of Columbia, and U.S. territories have the capacity to analyze TBI death and hospitalization data. This could be accomplished by continuing to fund TBI surveillance states and by increasing funding to Core injury surveillance states so that the Core states could expand their activities to include TBI surveillance. Combining Core injury surveillance and TBI surveillance into a single surveillance effort in each state was also recommended. (Note: Beginning in August 2005, CDC will fund approximately 30 states for a five-year cooperative agreement that combines Core injury and TBI surveillance (Program Announcement 05027: "Public Health Injury Surveillance and Prevention Program.")

2. CDC should decrease the lag time between identifying and reporting TBI surveillance data.

   ◦ Currently, lags of 12 to 18 months or greater occur before states have access to TBI data; CDC's review process further delays reporting of data. These lags should be reduced to the greatest extent possible.

3. CDC should facilitate consistency and comparability of data across TBI surveillance and research. This can be accomplished by working with other agencies, researchers, and experts to–

   ◦ Promote the use of a uniform TBI case definition.

   ◦ Encourage the use of all diagnosis fields in studies that identify TBI cases from hospitalization or emergency department data. Some studies identify cases only from the first-listed diagnosis. Using data from only one field excludes those with diagnoses listed in the other fields and underestimates the number of people with TBI.

- Develop a common taxonomy for collecting key surveillance and follow-up study data including:

  - Services used by people with TBI;
  - Severity, including the strengths and limitations of the ICDMAP computer program (which translates ICD-9-CM diagnosis codes into AIS codes and severity scores). (MacKenzie et al., 1989)
  - Outcomes (The National Center for Medical Rehabilitation Research [NCMRR] is developing definitions for research purposes as part of development of a Clinical Trials Network that may be useful for other studies. See the TBI Clinical Trials Network: www.tbi-ct.org);
  - Preexisting conditions, including previous TBI;
  - A standard definition for other trauma (the Barell Matrix may be useful; see www.cdc.gov/nchs/about/otheract/ice/barellmatrix.htm);
  - Recommended time intervals for collecting follow-up data;
  - Employment.

- Incorporate the information above into guidelines for conducting surveillance and collecting follow-up data; then, the guidelines should be widely disseminated. Guidelines should also apply to TBI data collection efforts not funded by CDC.

- National level

  1. CDC should continue to use existing national data sets to estimate the impact of TBI in the United States. (Note: Detailed national data were recently analyzed and published in a CDC report [Langlois et al., 2004].)

     - As part of this effort, CDC should evaluate the relative usefulness of the following national data sets maintained by the National Center for Health Statistics (NCHS) to determine their potential for monitoring TBI rates and trends in the U.S.:

       - National Vital Statistics System (NVSS)–mortality data
       - National Hospital Discharge Survey (NHDS)–hospital discharge data from a representative sample of U.S. hospitals

- National Hospital Ambulatory Medical Care Survey (NHAMCS)–data from a representative sample of hospital emergency departments
- National Health Interview Survey (NHIS)–data on the health status of a representative sample of U.S. residents obtained by telephone interview

For more information about NCHS data sets, see www.cdc.gov/nchs.

Identifying and Contacting People with TBI

1. CDC should consider ways to help develop and encourage comparable and consistent legislation within states.

2. CDC should help states interpret and apply provisions of the Health Insurance Portability and Accountability Act (HIPAA) to make sure surveillance and other TBI-related data collection efforts can continue, while maintaining confidentiality of the data.

Linking People with TBI to Services

CDC has funded several small pilot projects to explore the potential for using TBI surveillance data systems to link people with TBI to information about services.

1. CDC should support additional small linkage pilot projects in states. States that demonstrate effective linkage activities should receive ongoing support.

2. CDC should promote the development of linkages by conducting a workshop for states with interest and potential to conduct such data linkages. Participants should include:

- CDC grantees from states with experience conducting linkage projects;
- States interested in developing new linkage projects;
- Representatives of the National Association of State Head Injury Administrators (NASHIA);
- Brain Injury Association of America (BIAA) state affiliates;
- Grantees of the Health Resources and Services Administration (HRSA) TBI State Grant Program.

3. CDC should support the development, pilot testing, and evaluation of ways to link to services people with mild TBI and others who are not routinely identified or are missed by existing registries and surveillance programs.

4. CDC should facilitate development of a national linkage infrastructure by supporting the establishment of a national one-call information center with an 800 number that automatically connects callers to information and resources about TBI in their home states. (Note: CDC began implementing this effort in September 2004 by funding the Brain Injury Association of America to conduct a three-year pilot project.)

Follow-up Data Collection

- Children

CDC's highest priority should be to conduct follow-up studies to document long-term disability associated with TBI among children. Specifically, CDC should:

1. Fund a detailed follow-up study of school-age children, including children with mild TBI seen in an emergency department but not admitted to a hospital.

2. Consider collaborating with the U.S. Department of Education on a study to identify children with TBI in schools. The numbers of children with TBI reported by special education programs is much lower than would be expected based on the numbers of children who sustain a TBI each year; thus, better estimates are needed.

3. Explore the use of existing data sets for identifying children with TBI in schools.

4. Develop simplified follow-up methods for collecting information about TBI outcomes among children. These measures should apply in a wide range of settings.

5. Support research to develop methods and conduct studies that retrospectively identify children (and adults) with a prior diagnosis of TBI.

6. Build state capacity to conduct simplified follow-up data collection among school-age children with TBI. This would be facilitated by developing and publishing guidelines based on experience in conducting the follow-up study of TBI outcomes among school-age children described previously.

7. Fund research to develop methods for conducting follow-up studies of children younger than school age.

8. Monitor progress and provide input to the planned NIH National Children's Study (NCS) to include TBI as a topic of investigation. (Note: CDC staff participated in the planning and moderating of a meeting in September 2003 to discuss the potential for studying mild TBI in children as part of the NCS.)

9. Fund research on outcomes of sports-related injuries and intentional injuries among children.

- Adults

  1. CDC should evaluate the impact of the currently funded TBI follow-up study in South Carolina. The methods, findings, and lessons learned should be disseminated widely.

  2. CDC should develop simplified follow-up methods for application in a wide range of settings, especially health departments. These should be based on the methods developed for the Colorado and South Carolina follow-up studies.

3. Future follow-up studies should use new approaches to assessing health status (including the Short-Form-36 [SF-36] Health Survey [Medical Outcomes Trust, Inc., 20 Park Plaza, Suite 1014, Boston, Massachusetts 02116]). These new versions are administered by computer; they are based on patterns of response and reduce participants' response burden by eliminating the need to answer all questions.

4. CDC should help build state capacity to apply simplified follow-up methods that assess TBI outcomes among adults.

5. TBI researchers at CDC should learn more about disability measures being developed and used by other researchers:

   ◦ Communicate with researchers who develop participation measures and support or provide input to the development of such measure;

   ◦ Familiarize themselves with the International Classification of Function, Disability, and Health (ICF) (see www3.who.int/icf/icftemplate) and other developments in the disability research field.

Other Recommendations

Experts identified several other efforts which could advance the TBI field:

- Disability and other outcomes of TBI

  1. CDC should support research on the effects of aging on health among people already living with TBI-related disability.

  2. CDC should consider supporting research on mental health, depression, and post-traumatic stress disorder (PTSD) and their association with TBI.

  3. CDC should, in response to the Children's Health Act of 2000, support studies of the incidence of TBI and prevalence of TBI-related disability among people in institutions (i.e., nursing homes, psychiatric facilities, and prisons). (Note: As of January 2005, CDC has funded four pilot studies to identify people in prisons and nursing homes who have sustained a TBI.)

- Data linkage

  1. CDC should build state capacity to link TBI data to other data sets such as:

     ◦ Medicaid (includes nursing homes), Medicare, and other health payers;
     ◦ Special education;
     ◦ Vocational rehabilitation;
     ◦ Mental health;
     ◦ Social Security Administration;
     ◦ Juvenile/criminal justice systems;
     ◦ Foster care.

  2. CDC should develop a strategic plan for research that includes linking data from TBI data systems to other data sources. Linking these data could provide policy-relevant information, especially cost data, to support the need for increased state and federal funding for TBI services. Evidence about the cost of providing services compared with the cost of providing financial assistance to people who do not receive services can be very powerful in supporting the need for, and benefits of, services.

  3. CDC should consider holding a workshop for states with interest and potential to conduct such data linkages (e.g., state health department personnel, university-based researchers, and funding agencies). CDC staff could present potential research topics and methods for collecting policy relevant information.

  4. CDC should fund a study of states with registries that have been successful in developing state and federal resources for people with TBI to identify lessons learned regarding the use of data and other factors that might be useful to other states and TBI advocates. (Note: In 2003, CDC funded a small study to evaluate and report lessons learned from the Florida TBI registry and the results have been published in a peer-reviewed journal [Stuart 2004]).

5. CDC should explore the possibility of linking data sets used to track the costs of other disabling conditions to determine whether similar methods are applicable to tracking the costs of TBI.

6. CDC should support TBI research using qualitative research methods. These methods are particularly useful for evaluating programs and for investigating TBI-related issues that have not been thoroughly studied to inform methods for more detailed epidemiologic studies (Note: In 2000, CDC funded qualitative studies in Colorado [Sample 2004] and South Carolina [Leith 2004] to determine the feasibility of linking people with TBI in those states to information about services, and in Florida to determine the lessons learned from their TBI registry [Stuart 2004]. CDC also supported qualitative research to investigate violence among people with TBI. A peer-reviewed publication from this effort is in progress.)

- Collaboration with other agencies

Health Resources and Services Administration (HRSA)

1. CDC should continue collaborations between its grantees and grantees of the HRSA TBI Program. HRSA grantees are funded to develop the infrastructure for TBI services within their states. These collaborations will help HRSA grantees and state health department injury prevention personnel bridge the "cultural gap" between the injury prevention and long-term disability communities and help both organizations understand the mutual benefits of working together.

2. CDC should collaborate on TBI-related issues with the HRSA Emergency Medical Services for Children (EMSC) program. EMSC's goals are to ensure that state-of-the-art emergency medical care is available for all ill or injured children and adolescents; that pediatric services are well integrated into an emergency medical services (EMS) system; and that the entire spectrum of emergency services, including primary prevention of illness and injury, acute care, and rehabilitation, are provided to children and adolescents. A federal grant program supports state and local action. (For more detail see www.ask.hrsa.gov/orgdetail.cfm?id=252.)

American College of Surgeons (ACS)

1. CDC should collaborate with the American College of Surgeons' Committee on Trauma on TBI-related issues. This organization works to improve the care of injured and critically ill patients–before, en route to, and during hospitalization. (For more detail see: www.facs.org/about/corppro.html.)

Mild TBI

- Taxonomy

1. CDC should explore the potential for finding and promoting the use of an accurate term so that effective educational messages can be developed. "Mild" TBI refers to the severity of the injury to the brain itself at the time of initial diagnosis. Concussions are frequently described as mild TBIs. However, people with brain injuries that appear mild at the time of diagnosis can experience consequences that are not mild, including problems with memory, behavior, and emotional control. Studies are needed to show how the public currently perceives the term "mild TBI" so that educational messages describing the potential long-term consequences of mild TBI can be developed. Such studies will lay the groundwork for making sure people with long-term problems resulting from mild TBI are identified and are provided the services they need.

- Methods development

1. CDC should support research to develop accurate methods for identifying people with mild TBI. This includes developing an improved case definition for identifying people with mild TBI from administrative data sets, including CDC-funded TBI surveillance of TBIs treated in hospital emergency departments. See the TBI Report to Congress on Mild Traumatic Brain Injury in the United States: www.cdc.gov/doc.do/id/0900f3ec8006b2e5). (Note: Beginning September 2004, CDC funded two TBI surveillance states [South Carolina and New York] to conduct a study to validate an improved ICD-9-CM code-based case definition to identify people with mild TBI from administrative data sets.

In a similar effort, with CDC funding, the Michigan Public Health Institute is currently evaluating the level of agreement between two approaches to identifying non-hospitalized cases of mild TBI treated in emergency departments using a surveillance ICD-9-CM case definition vs. using a prospective case identification protocol.)

- Data collection

    1. CDC should maintain current state-based surveillance of TBIs treated in hospital emergency departments (ED) to track declines in TBI hospitalization rates and report data on the portion of the population with mild TBI that is identified in emergency department data sets. These data sets also include important information about TBI among children since approximately 10 times as many TBIs among children are seen in emergency departments as are admitted to hospitals. (Note: ED data for TBI from the National Hospital Ambulatory Care Survey [NHAMCS] were recently analyzed and published in a CDC report [Langlois et al., 2004]. CDC has also funded a pilot study to determine the feasibility of using injury data from the Consumer Product Safety Commission's National Electronic Injury Surveillance System [NEISS] to identify TBIs treated in the ED.)

    2. CDC should fund studies of the long-term outcomes of mild TBI among people treated in emergency departments to document that for some people with mild TBI, the effects of the TBI are not mild.

- Education

    1. CDC should conduct research to develop effective messages to educate healthcare providers and the public that TBIs that are initially diagnosed as mild do not always result in mild consequences. Although most patients with concussions or mild TBIs do appear to recover fully from their injuries, some experience long-term memory, emotional or other problems that can adversely affect their potential to work and perform daily activities.

2. CDC, state Brain Injury Associations, and other organizations should work with hospital associations and emergency medical and trauma systems to provide information about mild TBI routinely with discharge orders (e.g., by storing information and printing it along with discharge instructions to be given to emergency department patients diagnosed with TBI).

Summary

By definition, TBI surveillance and registries differ, but many of the functions that registries serve could be implemented by enhancing existing surveillance systems. Leveraging existing TBI and injury data collection efforts, including TBI surveillance that is already ongoing in states, would result in greater efficiency and cost savings than developing a new registry-type data collection system.

References

Brooks CA, Gabella B, Hoffman R, Sosin D, Whiteneck G. Traumatic brain injury: designing and implementing a population-based follow-up system. *Archives of Physical Medicine & Rehabilitation* 1997;78:S26–30.

Feinstein AR. Clinical Epidemiology: The Architecture of Clinical Research. Philadelphia: WB Saunders; 1998.

Foege WH, Hogan RC, Newton LH. Surveillance projects for selected diseases. *International Journal of Epidemiology* 1976;5:29–37.

General Accounting Office. Traumatic Brain Injury: Programs Supporting Long-term Services in Selected States. Report #GAO/HEHS-98-55. Washington (DC): U.S. General Accounting Office, Health Education and Human Services Division; 1998.

Langlois JA, Kegler SR, Butler JA, Gotsch KE, Johnson RL, Reichard AA, Webb KW, Coronado VG, Selassie AW, Thurman DJ. Traumatic brain injury-related hospital discharges: results from a 14-state surveillance system, 1997. *MMWR Surveillance Summaries* 2003;52(No. SS-4):1–20.

Langlois JA, Rutland-Brown W, Thomas KE: *Traumatic Brain Injury in the United States: Emergency Department Visits, Hospitalizations, and Deaths.* Atlanta (GA): Centers for Disease Control and Prevention, National Center for Injury Prevention and Control; 2004.

Leith KH, Phillips L, Sample PL. Exploring the service needs and experiences of persons with TBI and their families: the South Carolina experience. *Brain Injury* 2004;18:1191-1208.

MacKenzie EJ, Steinwachs DM, Shankar B. Classifying trauma severity based on hospital discharge diagnosis. *Medical Care.* 1989;27(4):412–422.

Marr A, Coronado V, editors. Central Nervous System Injury Surveillance: Annual Data Submission Standards for the Year 2002. Atlanta: U.S. Department of Health and Human Services, CDC, National Center for Injury Prevention and Control; 2004.

National Center for Injury Prevention and Control. Report and Recommendations from the Traumatic Brain Injury in Public Health Meeting. Atlanta: U.S. Department of Health and Human Services, CDC, National Center for Injury Prevention and Control; 1999a.

National Center for Injury Prevention and Control. Traumatic Brain Injury in the United States: A Report to Congress. Atlanta: U.S. Department of Health and Human Services, CDC, National Center for Injury Prevention and Control; 1999b.

National Institutes of Health. Consequences of traumatic brain injury. In: NIH. Report of the Consensus Development Conference on the Rehabilitation of Persons with Traumatic Brain Injury. Bethesda (MD): U.S. Department of Health and Human Services, NIH; 1999. p. 169–202.

Pickelsimer E, Gu J, Gravelle W, Selassie A, Langlois J. Population-based follow-up of persons with traumatic brain injury: the South Carolina Traumatic Brain Injury Follow-up System. *Brain Injury Source* 2002;6:18–20.

Sample PL, Johns N, Gabella B, Langlois J. Can traumatic brain injury surveillance systems be used to link individuals with TBI to services? *Brain Injury* 2004;18:1177-1189.

State and Territorial Injury Prevention Directors' Association. Safe States, 2003 Edition. Atlanta: State and Territorial Injury Prevention Directors' Association; 2003.

Stuart M. Fighting the silent epidemic: The Florida Brain and Spinal Cord Injury Program. *Journal of Head Trauma Rehabilitation* 2004;19:329-340.

Thurman DJ, Alverson C, Dunn KA, Guerrero J, Sniezek JE. Traumatic brain injury in the United States: a public health perspective. *Journal of Head Trauma Rehabilitation* 1999;14:602–15.

Appendix 1

**Additional Resources: Articles and Book Chapters
about Surveillance and Registries**

Harrison C, Dijkers M. Traumatic brain injury registries in the United States: an overview.
Brain Injury 1992;6:203–12.

Parrish RG II, McDonnel S. Sources of health-related information. In: Teutsch S, Churchill RE,
editors. Principles and Practice of Public Health Surveillance. New York: Oxford University
Press; 2000. p. 30–75.

Solomon D, Henry R, Hogan J, Van Amburg G, Taylor J. Evaluation and implementation of
public health registries. *Public Health Reports* 1991;106:142–50.

Wedell J. Registers and registries: a review. *International Journal of Epidemiology*
1973;2:221–28.

Appendix 2

Websites by Topic

TBI Registries

Florida Brain and Spinal Cord Injury Program (BSCIP)
    www.doh.state.fl.us/Workforce/BrainSC

SC Traumatic Brain Injury Follow-up Registry
    sctbifr.musc.edu

Virginia TBI Registry
    www.biav.net/central_registry.htm

Defense and Veterans Brain Injury Center (DVBIC)
    www.dvbic.org

CDC TBI and State Injury Programs and Projects

TBI Data Systems
    www.cdc.gov/ncipc/profiles/tbi

Core State Injury Program
    www.cdc.gov/ncipc/profiles/core_state

Injury Indicators
    www.cdc.gov/ncipc/pub-res/indicators

CDC's National Program of Cancer Registries

www.cdc.gov/cancer/npcr

TBI Legislation Authorizing CDC's TBI Activities

PL 104-166: The Traumatic Brain Injury Act of 1996

http://thomas.loc.gov/bss/d104/d104laws.html. Select the range 104-151 to 104-200 and click search. Scroll down to 166. Select text or pdf.

HR 4365: The Children's Health Act of 2000

http://thomas.loc.gov/cgi-bin/bdquery/z?d106:HR04365:. Select text or pdf.

Appendix 3

Other Websites

American College of Surgeons
www.facs.org/about/corppro.html

Barell Injury Matrix
www.cdc.gov/nchs/about/otheract/ice/barellmatrix.htm

Brain Injury Association of America
www.biausa.org

Health Resources and Services Administration: Emergency Medical Services for Children Program
www.ask.hrsa.gov/orgdetail.cfm?id=252

Health Resources and Services Administration: TBI Grant Program
www.tbitac.org

International Classification of Diseases, Health, and Disability
www3.who.int/icf/icftemplate

National Association of State Head Injury Administrators (NASHIA)
Guide to State Government Brain Injury Polices, Funding, and Services
Chapter on Data Collection (p. 38–47)
www.nashia.org/pdocfiles/RC/reguide.htm

National Center for Medical Rehabilitation Research, TBI Clinical Trials Network
www.tbi-ct.org